Copyright © 2023 by Monica Dimitrios

All rights reserved. No part of this publication may be reproduced, distributed, or transmitted in any form or by any means, including photocopying, recording, or other electronic or mechanical methods, without the prior written permission of the publisher, except in the case of brief quotations embodied in critical reviews and certain other noncommercial uses permitted by copyright law.

Table of Contents

NEUROPATHY

Peripheral neuropathy, a result of damage to the nerves located outside of the brain and spinal cord (peripheral nerves), often causes weakness, numbness and pain, usually in the hands and feet. It can also affect other areas and body functions including digestion, urination and circulation.

NEUROPATHY RECIPES

1. One-Pot Garlicky Shrimp & Broccoli

Prep Time: 20 mins

Total Time: 20 mins

Servings: 4

Ingredients

- 3 tablespoons extra-virgin olive oil, divided
- 6 medium cloves garlic, sliced, divided
- 4 cups small broccoli florets
- ½ cup diced red bell pepper
- ½ teaspoon salt, divided
- ½ teaspoon ground pepper, divided
- 1 pound peeled and deveined raw shrimp (21-30 count)
- 2 teaspoons lemon juice, plus more to taste

Directions

1. Heat 2 tablespoons oil in a large saucepan over medium heat. Add half the garlic and cook until beginning to brown, about 1 minute. Add broccoli, bell pepper and 1/4 teaspoon each salt and pepper.

Cover and cook, stirring once or twice and adding 1 tablespoon water if the pot is too dry, until the vegetables are tender, 3 to 5 minutes. Transfer to a bowl and keep warm.

2. Increase heat to medium-high and add the remaining 1 tablespoon oil to the pot. Add the remaining garlic and cook until beginning to brown, about 1 minute. Add shrimp and the remaining 1/4 teaspoon each salt and pepper; cook, stirring, until the shrimp are just cooked through, 3 to 5 minutes. Return the broccoli mixture to the pot along with lemon juice and stir to combine.

Prep Time: 20 mins

Total Time: 20 mins

Servings: 4

Ingredients

- 1 pound chicken cutlets
- ¼ teaspoon salt, divided
- ¼ teaspoon ground pepper, divided
- ½ cup slivered oil-packed sun-dried tomatoes, plus 1 tablespoon oil from the jar
- ½ cup finely chopped shallots
- ½ cup dry white wine
- ½ cup heavy cream
- 2 tablespoons chopped fresh parsley

Directions

1. Sprinkle chicken with 1/8 teaspoon each salt and pepper. Heat sun-dried tomato oil in a large skillet over medium heat. Add the chicken and cook, turning once, until browned and an instant-read thermometer inserted into the thickest part

registers 165°F, about 6 minutes total. Transfer to a plate.

2. Add sun-dried tomatoes and shallots to the pan. Cook, stirring, for 1 minute. Increase heat to high and add wine. Cook, scraping up any browned bits, until the liquid has mostly evaporated, about 2 minutes. Reduce heat to medium and stir in cream, any accumulated juices from the chicken and the remaining 1/8 teaspoon each salt and pepper; simmer for 2 minutes. Return the chicken to the pan and turn to coat with the sauce. Serve the chicken topped with the sauce and parsley.

3. Cheesy Ground Beef & Cauliflower Casserole

Prep Time: 30 mins

Total Time: 30 mins

Servings: 6

Ingredients

- 1 tablespoon extra-virgin olive oil
- ½ cup chopped onion
- 1 medium green bell pepper, chopped
- 1 pound lean ground beef
- 3 cups bite-size cauliflower florets
- 3 cloves garlic, minced
- 2 tablespoons chili powder
- 2 teaspoons ground cumin
- 1 teaspoon dried oregano
- ½ teaspoon salt
- ¼ teaspoon ground chipotle
- 1 (15 ounce) can no-salt-added petite-diced tomatoes
- 2 cups shredded extra-sharp Cheddar cheese
- ⅓ cup sliced pickled jalapeños

Directions

1. Position rack in upper third of oven. Preheat broiler to high.

2. Heat oil in a large oven-safe skillet over medium heat. Add onion and bell pepper; cook, stirring, until softened, about 5 minutes. Add beef and cauliflower; cook, stirring and breaking the beef up into smaller pieces, until it is no longer pink, 5 to 7 minutes. Stir in garlic, chili powder, cumin, oregano, salt and chipotle; cook until fragrant, about 1 minute. Add tomatoes and their juices; bring to a simmer and cook, stirring occasionally, until liquid is reduced and the cauliflower is tender, about 3 minutes more. Remove from heat.

3. Sprinkle cheese over the beef mixture and top with sliced jalapeños. Broil until the cheese is melted and browned in spots, 2 to 3 minutes.

Prep Time: 15 mins

Total Time: 50 mins

Servings: 12

Ingredients

- 3 cups old-fashioned rolled oats
- 1 ¼ cups low-fat milk
- ½ cup unsweetened applesauce
- ⅓ cup packed light brown sugar
- 1 tablespoon grated lemon zest
- ¼ cup lemon juice
- 2 large eggs, lightly beaten
- 1 teaspoon baking powder
- 1 teaspoon vanilla extract
- ½ teaspoon salt
- 1 cup frozen blueberries, preferably wild

Directions

1. Preheat oven to 375°F. Coat a muffin tin with cooking spray.

2. Combine oats, milk, applesauce, brown sugar, lemon zest, lemon juice, eggs, baking powder, vanilla and salt in a large bowl. Fold in frozen blueberries. Divide the mixture among the prepared muffin cups, about 1/3 cup each. Bake until a toothpick inserted in the center comes out clean, about 25 minutes.

3. Cool in the pan for 10 to 15 minutes, then turn out onto a wire rack. Serve warm or at room temperature.

5. Weight-Loss Cabbage Soup

Prep Time: 35 mins

Total Time: 55 mins

Servings: 6

Ingredients

- 2 tablespoons extra-virgin olive oil
- 1 medium onion, chopped
- 2 medium carrots, chopped
- 2 stalks celery, chopped
- 1 medium red bell pepper, chopped
- 2 cloves garlic, minced
- 1 ½ teaspoons Italian seasoning
- ½ teaspoon ground pepper
- ¼ teaspoon salt
- 8 cups low-sodium vegetable broth
- 1 medium head green cabbage, halved and sliced
- 1 large tomato, chopped
- 2 teaspoons white-wine vinegar

Directions

1. Heat oil in a large pot over medium heat. Add onion, carrots and celery. Cook, stirring, until the vegetables begin to soften, 6 to 8 minutes. Add bell pepper, garlic, Italian seasoning, pepper and salt and cook, stirring, for 2 minutes.

2. Add broth, cabbage and tomato; increase heat to medium-high and bring to a boil. Reduce heat to maintain a simmer, partially cover and cook until all the vegetables are tender, 15 to 20 minutes more. Remove from heat and stir in vinegar.

Prep Time: 15 mins

Total Time: 20 mins

Servings: 6

Ingredients

- 1 medium serrano pepper, cut into thirds
- 4 large cloves garlic
- 1 2-inch piece fresh ginger, peeled and coarsely chopped
- 1 medium yellow onion, chopped (1-inch)
- 6 tablespoons canola oil or grapeseed oil
- 2 teaspoons ground coriander
- 2 teaspoons ground cumin
- ½ teaspoon ground turmeric
- 2 ¼ cups no-salt-added canned diced tomatoes with their juice (from a 28-ounce can)
- ¾ teaspoon kosher salt
- 2 15-ounce cans chickpeas, rinsed
- 2 teaspoons garam masala
- Fresh cilantro for garnish

Directions

1. Pulse serrano, garlic and ginger in a food processor until minced. Scrape down the sides and pulse again. Add onion; pulse until finely chopped, but not watery.

2. Heat oil in a large saucepan over medium-high heat. Add the onion mixture and cook, stirring occasionally, until softened, 3 to 5 minutes. Add coriander, cumin and turmeric and cook, stirring, for 2 minutes.

3. Pulse tomatoes in the food processor until finely chopped. Add to the pan along with salt. Reduce heat to maintain a simmer and cook, stirring occasionally, for 4 minutes. Add chickpeas and garam masala, reduce heat to a gentle simmer, cover and cook, stirring occasionally, for 5 minutes more. Serve topped with cilantro, if desired.

7. Baked Banana-Nut Oatmeal Cups

Prep Time: 15 mins

Total Time: 50 mins

Servings: 12

Ingredients

- 3 cups rolled oats
- 1 ½ cups low-fat milk
- 2 ripe bananas, mashed (about 3/4 cup)
- ⅓ cup packed brown sugar
- 2 large eggs, lightly beaten
- 1 teaspoon baking powder
- 1 teaspoon ground cinnamon
- 1 teaspoon vanilla extract
- ½ teaspoon salt
- ½ cup toasted chopped pecans

Directions

1. Preheat oven to 375°F. Coat a muffin tin with cooking spray.
2. Combine oats, milk, bananas, brown sugar, eggs, baking powder, cinnamon, vanilla and salt in a

large bowl. Fold in pecans. Divide the mixture among the muffin cups (about 1/3 cup each). Bake until a toothpick inserted in the center comes out clean, about 25 minutes. Cool in the pan for 10 minutes, then turn out onto a wire rack. Serve warm or at room temperature.

8. Breakfast Peanut Butter-Chocolate Chip Oatmeal Cakes

Prep Time: 15 mins

Total Time: 50 mins

Servings: 12

Ingredients

- 3 cups old-fashioned rolled oats
- 1 ½ cups low-fat milk
- ½ cup creamy natural peanut butter, divided
- ¼ cup unsweetened applesauce
- 2 large eggs, lightly beaten
- 3 tablespoons packed light brown sugar
- 1 teaspoon baking powder
- 1 teaspoon vanilla extract
- ½ teaspoon salt
- ¼ cup mini semisweet chocolate chips

Directions

1. Preheat oven to 375°F. Coat a 12-cup muffin tin with cooking spray.

2. Combine oats, milk, 1/4 cup peanut butter, applesauce, eggs, brown sugar, baking powder, vanilla and salt in a large bowl. Fill each muffin cup with a heaping 2 tablespoons of batter, then divide the remaining 1/4 cup peanut butter and chocolate chips among the muffin cups, about 1 teaspoon each. Cover with the remaining batter, about 2 tablespoons each. Bake until a toothpick inserted in the center comes out clean, about 25 minutes. Cool in the pan for 10 minutes, then turn out onto a wire rack. Serve warm or at room temperature.

9. Melting Potatoes

Prep Time: 25 mins

Total Time: 1 hr 10 mins

Servings: 6

Ingredients

- 2 pounds Yukon Gold potatoes, peeled and cut into 1-inch slices
- 2 tablespoons butter, melted
- 2 tablespoons extra-virgin olive oil
- 2 teaspoons chopped fresh thyme
- 1 teaspoon chopped fresh rosemary
- ¾ teaspoon salt
- ½ teaspoon ground pepper
- 1 cup low-sodium vegetable broth or chicken broth
- 5 cloves garlic, peeled and smashed

Directions

1. Position rack in upper third of oven; preheat to 500°F.
2. Toss potatoes, butter, oil, thyme, rosemary, salt and pepper in a large bowl. Arrange in a single

layer in a 9-by-13-inch metal baking pan. (Do not use a glass dish, which could shatter.) Roast, flipping once, until browned, about 30 minutes.

3. Carefully add broth and garlic to the pan. Continue roasting until most of the broth is absorbed and the potatoes are very tender, about 15 minutes more. Serve hot.

Prep Time: 25 mins

Total Time: 1 hr 5 mins

Servings: 6

Ingredients

- 2 tablespoons extra-virgin olive oil
- 8 ounces sliced fresh mixed wild mushrooms such as cremini, shiitake, button and/or oyster mushrooms
- 1 ½ cups thinly sliced sweet onion
- 1 tablespoon thinly sliced garlic
- 5 ounces fresh baby spinach (about 8 cups), coarsely chopped
- 6 large eggs
- ¼ cup whole milk
- ¼ cup half-and-half
- 1 tablespoon Dijon mustard
- 1 tablespoon fresh thyme leaves, plus more for garnish
- ¼ teaspoon salt
- ¼ teaspoon ground pepper

- 1 ½ cups shredded Gruyère cheese

Directions

1. Preheat oven to 375 degrees F. Coat a 9-inch pie pan with cooking spray; set aside.

2. Heat oil in a large nonstick skillet over medium-high heat; swirl to coat the pan. Add mushrooms; cook, stirring occasionally, until browned and tender, about 8 minutes. Add onion and garlic; cook, stirring often, until softened and tender, about 5 minutes. Add spinach; cook, tossing constantly, until wilted, 1 to 2 minutes. Remove from heat.

3. Whisk eggs, milk, half-and-half, mustard, thyme, salt and pepper in a medium bowl. Fold in the mushroom mixture and cheese. Spoon into the prepared pie pan. Bake until set and golden brown, about 30 minutes. Let stand for 10 minutes; slice. Garnish with thyme and serve.

11. Chicken & Spinach Skillet Pasta with Lemon &
Parmesan

Prep Time: 25 mins

Total Time: 25 mins

Servings: 4

Ingredients

- 8 ounces gluten-free penne pasta or whole-wheat penne pasta
- 2 tablespoons extra-virgin olive oil
- 1 pound boneless, skinless chicken breast or thighs, trimmed, if necessary, and cut into bite-size pieces
- ½ teaspoon salt
- ¼ teaspoon ground pepper
- 4 cloves garlic, minced
- ½ cup dry white wine
- Juice and zest of 1 lemon
- 10 cups chopped fresh spinach
- 4 tablespoons grated Parmesan cheese, divided

Directions

1. Cook pasta according to package directions. Drain and set aside.

2. Meanwhile, heat oil in a large high-sided skillet over medium-high heat. Add chicken, salt and pepper; cook, stirring occasionally, until just cooked through, 5 to 7 minutes. Add garlic and cook, stirring, until fragrant, about 1 minute. Stir in wine, lemon juice and zest; bring to a simmer.

3. Remove from heat. Stir in spinach and the cooked pasta. Cover and let stand until the spinach is just wilted. Divide among 4 plates and top each serving with 1 tablespoon Parmesan.

12. Cinnamon-Roll Overnight Oats

Prep Time: 5 mins

Total Time: 8 hrs

Servings: 5

Ingredients

- 2 1/2 cups old-fashioned rolled oats
- 2 1/2 cups unsweetened nondairy milk, such as almond or coconut
- 6 teaspoons light brown sugar
- 1 ½ teaspoons vanilla extract
- 1 ¼ teaspoons ground cinnamon
- ½ teaspoon salt

Directions

1. Stir oats, milk, brown sugar, vanilla, cinnamon and salt together in a large bowl. Divide among five 8-ounce jars. Screw on lids and refrigerate overnight or for up to 5 days.

13. Loaded Cauliflower Casserole

Prep Time: 20 mins

Total Time: 1 hr

Servings: 8

Ingredients

- 3 slices bacon
- 1 head cauliflower (about 2 pounds), cut into bite-size pieces
- ½ teaspoon ground pepper
- ¼ teaspoon salt
- 1 ¼ cups shredded sharp Cheddar cheese, divided
- ⅔ cup sour cream
- 4 scallions, sliced, divided

Directions

1. Preheat oven to 425°F.
2. Place bacon in a large nonstick skillet over medium heat; cook until crisp, 6 to 8 minutes. Transfer to a paper-towel-lined plate and let cool. (Reserve the drippings in the pan.)

3. Combine cauliflower, pepper, salt and the bacon drippings in a 9-by-13-inch baking dish. Roast, stirring twice, until tender, about 35 minutes.

4. Meanwhile, combine 1 cup cheese, 2/3 cup sour cream and half the scallions in a small bowl. When the cauliflower is tender, stir the cheese mixture into the cauliflower in the pan. Sprinkle with the remaining 1/4 cup cheese. Bake until hot, 5 to 7 minutes more.

5. Chop the cooled bacon. Sprinkle the hot casserole with the bacon and the remaining scallions.

14. Twice-Baked Potatoes Casserole

Prep Time: 15 mins

Total Time: 1 hr

Servings: 12

Ingredients

- 3 pounds medium russet potatoes, scrubbed
- 1 teaspoon extra-virgin olive oil
- ⅓ cup reduced-fat cream cheese
- ¼ cup sour cream
- 1 ½ cups whole milk
- 1 ½ cups shredded sharp Cheddar cheese, divided
- 5 slices bacon, cooked and crumbled, divided
- ¼ cup thinly sliced scallions, plus more for garnish
- ¾ teaspoon salt
- ½ teaspoon ground pepper

Directions

1. Preheat oven to 400°F and line a large rimmed baking sheet with foil. Rub potatoes with oil and pierce all over with a fork. Place on the prepared baking sheet. Bake until tender, about 1 hour.

(Alternatively, to microwave, pierce potatoes all over with a fork and place on a large microwave-safe plate, omitting the oil. Microwave on High until tender, about 20 minutes.) Let cool slightly, abut 10 minutes.

2. Meanwhile, whisk cream cheese and sour cream together in a medium bowl until smooth; gradually whisk in milk until well incorporated.

3. Coat a 9-by-13-inch ceramic baking dish with cooking spray. Cut the potatoes in half lengthwise and roughly chop the halves. Place the chopped potatoes in a large bowl and, using a potato masher, mash until mostly smooth. Gradually add the milk mixture, stirring just until incorporated. Add 1/2 cup Cheddar, 1/4 cup bacon, scallions, salt and pepper; stir until well combined. Transfer the mixture to the prepared baking dish. Sprinkle with the remaining 1 cup Cheddar.

4. Bake until the cheese is melted and the edges are browned, about 25 minutes. Sprinkle with the

remaining bacon. Garnish with scallions, if
desired.

15. Salmon-Stuffed Avocados

Prep Time: 15 mins

Total Time: 15 mins

Servings: 4

Ingredients

- ½ cup nonfat plain Greek yogurt
- ½ cup diced celery
- 2 tablespoons chopped fresh parsley
- 1 tablespoon lime juice
- 2 teaspoons mayonnaise
- 1 teaspoon Dijon mustard
- ⅛ teaspoon salt
- ⅛ teaspoon ground pepper
- 2 (5 ounce) cans salmon, drained, flaked, skin and bones removed
- 2 avocados
- Chopped chives for garnish

Directions

1. Combine yogurt, celery, parsley, lime juice, mayonnaise, mustard, salt, and pepper in a medium bowl; mix well. Add salmon and mix well.
2. Halve avocados lengthwise and remove pits. Scoop about 1 tablespoon flesh from each avocado half into a small bowl. Mash the scooped-out avocado flesh with a fork and stir into the salmon mixture.
3. Fill each avocado half with about 1/4 cup of the salmon mixture, mounding it on top of the avocado halves. Garnish with chives, if desired.

Prep Time: 10 mins

Total Time: 40 mins

Servings: 4

Ingredients

- 1 pound baby Yukon Gold potatoes, halved
- 2 tablespoons extra-virgin olive oil, divided
- ¾ teaspoon salt, divided
- ½ teaspoon ground pepper, divided
- 12 ounces asparagus, trimmed
- 2 tablespoons melted butter
- 1 tablespoon lemon juice
- 2 cloves garlic, minced
- 1 ¼ pounds salmon fillet, skinned and cut into 4 portions
- Chopped parsley for garnish

Directions

1. Preheat oven to 400 degrees F. Toss potatoes, 1 tablespoon oil, 1/4 teaspoon salt and 1/8 teaspoon

pepper together in a medium bowl. Spread in an even layer on a large rimmed baking sheet. Roast until starting to soften and brown, about 15 minutes.

2. Meanwhile, toss asparagus with the remaining 1 tablespoon oil, 1/8 teaspoon salt and 1/8 teaspoon pepper in the medium bowl. Combine butter, lemon juice, garlic, 1/4 teaspoon salt and the remaining 1/4 teaspoon pepper in a small bowl.

3. Sprinkle salmon with the remaining 1/8 teaspoon salt. Move the potatoes to one side of the pan. Place the salmon in the center of the pan; drizzle with the butter mixture. Spread the asparagus on the empty side of the pan. Roast until the salmon is just cooked through and the vegetables are tender, 10 to 12 minutes. Garnish with parsley.

Prep Time: 25 mins

Total Time: 50 mins

Servings: 6

Ingredients

- 2 tablespoons extra-virgin olive oil
- ¾ cup diced onion
- ¼ teaspoon salt, divided
- 1 medium red bell pepper, diced
- 1 tablespoon finely chopped fresh oregano
- 8 large eggs
- ¾ cup crumbled feta cheese
- ½ cup low-fat milk
- ½ teaspoon ground pepper
- 2 cups chopped fresh spinach
- ¼ cup sliced Kalamata olives

Directions

1. Preheat oven to 325 degrees F. Liberally coat a 12-cup muffin tin with cooking spray.

2. Heat oil in a large skillet over medium heat. Add onion and 1/8 teaspoon salt; cook, stirring, until starting to soften, about 3 minutes. Add bell pepper and oregano; cook, stirring, until the vegetables are tender and starting to brown, 4 to 5 minutes more. Remove from heat and let cool for 5 minutes.

3. Whisk eggs, feta, milk, pepper and the remaining 1/8 teaspoon salt in a large bowl. Stir in spinach, olives and the vegetable mixture. Divide among the prepared muffin cups.

4. Bake until firm to the touch, about 25 minutes. Let stand for 5 minutes before removing from the tin.

Prep Time: 35 mins

Total Time: 1 hr

Servings: 8

Ingredients

- 3 tablespoons extra-virgin olive oil, divided
- 1 pound lean ground beef
- 1 cup chopped onion
- 3 cloves garlic, minced
- 2 cups low-sodium chicken or beef broth
- 1 (15 ounce) can no-salt-added tomato sauce
- 1 cup long-grain white rice
- ½ teaspoon salt, divided
- ½ teaspoon ground pepper, divided
- 8 cups chopped green cabbage (1 1/4 pounds)
- 2 teaspoons dried dill
- ¼ teaspoon crushed red pepper
- 1 ½ cups shredded Cheddar cheese

Directions

1. Preheat oven to 350°F. Lightly coat a 9-by-13-inch baking dish with cooking spray.

2. Heat 1 tablespoon oil in a large saucepan over medium heat. Add ground beef and onion; cook, stirring, until the beef is no longer pink, about 5 minutes. Add garlic and cook until fragrant, about 1 minute. Stir in broth, tomato sauce, rice, 1/4 teaspoon salt and 1/4 teaspoon pepper; bring to a simmer. Cover, reduce heat to maintain a simmer and cook, stirring once or twice, until the rice is tender, about 17 minutes (the mixture will be a little saucy). Uncover and remove from heat.

3. Meanwhile, heat the remaining 2 tablespoons oil in a large skillet over medium heat. Add cabbage, dill, crushed red pepper and the remaining 1/4 teaspoon each salt and pepper. Cook, stirring, until the cabbage is just tender, 5 to 7 minutes. Remove from heat.

4. Spread half the cabbage in the bottom of the prepared baking dish. Top with half the beef mixture then half the cheese. Repeat with the

remaining cabbage, beef mixture and cheese. Bake until hot and the cheese has melted and started to brown, about 25 minutes.

Prep Time: 20 mins

Total Time: 20 mins

Servings: 4

Ingredients

- 1 (7 ounce) jar roasted red peppers, rinsed
- ¼ cup slivered almonds
- 4 tablespoons extra-virgin olive oil, divided
- 1 small clove garlic, minced
- 1 teaspoon paprika
- ½ teaspoon ground cumin
- ¼ teaspoon crushed red pepper
- 2 cups cooked quinoa
- ¼ cup Kalamata olives, chopped
- ¼ cup finely chopped red onion
- 1 (15 ounce) can chickpeas, rinsed
- 1 cup diced cucumber
- ¼ cup crumbled feta cheese
- 2 tablespoons finely chopped fresh parsley

Directions

1. Place peppers, almonds, 2 tablespoons oil, garlic, paprika, cumin and crushed red pepper (if using) in a mini food processor. Puree until fairly smooth.

2. Combine quinoa, olives, red onion and the remaining 2 tablespoons oil in a medium bowl.

3. To serve, divide the quinoa mixture among 4 bowls and top with equal amounts of the chickpeas, cucumber and the red pepper sauce. Sprinkle with feta and parsley.

20. Sweet Potato & Black Bean Chili

Prep Time: 25 mins

Total Time: 40 mins

Servings: 4

Ingredients

- 1 tablespoon plus 2 teaspoons extra-virgin olive oil
- 1 medium-large sweet potato, peeled and diced
- 1 large onion, diced
- 4 cloves garlic, minced
- 2 tablespoons chili powder
- 4 teaspoons ground cumin
- ½ teaspoon ground chipotle chile
- ¼ teaspoon salt
- 2 ½ cups water
- 2 15-ounce cans black beans, rinsed
- 1 14-ounce can diced tomatoes
- 4 teaspoons lime juice
- ½ cup chopped fresh cilantro

Directions

1. Heat oil in a Dutch oven over medium-high heat. Add sweet potato and onion and cook, stirring often, until the onion is beginning to soften, about 4 minutes. Add garlic, chili powder, cumin, chipotle and salt and cook, stirring constantly, for 30 seconds. Add water and bring to a simmer. Cover, reduce heat to maintain a gentle simmer and cook until the sweet potato is tender, 10 to 12 minutes.

2. Add beans, tomatoes and lime juice; increase heat to high and return to a simmer, stirring often. Reduce heat and simmer until slightly reduced, about 5 minutes. Remove from heat and stir in cilantro.

21. Lemon-Garlic Vinaigrette

Prep Time: 5 mins

Total Time: 5 mins

Servings: 10

Ingredients

- ¾ cup extra-virgin olive oil
- 5 tablespoons red-wine vinegar
- 3 tablespoons lemon juice
- 1 ½ tablespoons Dijon mustard
- 1 clove garlic, grated
- ¾ teaspoon salt
- Ground pepper to taste

Directions

1. Combine olive oil, vinegar, lemon juice, mustard, garlic, salt and pepper in a jar with a tight-fitting lid. Shake until well blended.

22. One-Pot Lentil & Vegetable Soup with Parmesan

Prep Time: 15 mins

Total Time: 40 mins

Servings: 6

Ingredients

- 2 tablespoons extra-virgin olive oil
- 3 cups fresh or frozen chopped onion, carrot and celery mix
- 4 cloves garlic, chopped
- 4 cups low-sodium vegetable or chicken broth
- 1 ½ cups green or brown lentils
- 1 (15-ounce) can unsalted diced tomatoes, undrained
- 2 teaspoons finely chopped fresh thyme
- ½ teaspoon salt
- ½ teaspoon ground pepper
- ½ teaspoon crushed red pepper
- ½ cup grated Parmesan cheese
- Parmesan rind
- 3 cups packed roughly chopped lacinato kale
- 1 ½ tablespoons red-wine vinegar

- Chopped fresh flat-leaf parsley for garnish

Directions

1. Heat oil in a Dutch oven or large pot over medium heat. Add onion, carrot and celery mix; cook, stirring occasionally, until softened, 6 to 10 minutes. Add garlic; cook, stirring often, until fragrant, about 30 seconds.

2. Stir in broth, lentils, tomatoes, thyme, salt, pepper, crushed red pepper and Parmesan rind, if using. Bring to a boil over medium-high heat. Reduce heat to medium-low; cover and cook, stirring occasionally, until the lentils are almost tender, 15 to 25 minutes, adding water as needed to thin to desired consistency.

3. Stir in kale. Cook, covered, until the kale is tender, 5 to 10 minutes. Remove and discard the Parmesan rind, if using. Stir in vinegar. Divide the soup among 6 bowls; sprinkle with Parmesan. Garnish with parsley, if desired.

23. Peanut Butter Energy Balls

Prep Time: 20 mins

Total Time: 20 mins

Servings: 17

Ingredients

- 2 cups rolled oats
- 1 cup natural peanut butter or other nut butter
- ½ cup honey
- ¼ cup mini chocolate chips
- ¼ cup unsweetened shredded coconut

Directions

1. Combine oats, peanut butter (or other nut butter), honey, chocolate chips and coconut in a medium bowl; stir well. Using a 1-tablespoon measure, roll the mixture into balls.

24. Black Bean-Quinoa Bowl

Prep Time: 10 mins

Total Time: 10 mins

Servings: 1

Ingredients

- ¾ cup canned black beans, rinsed
- ⅔ cup cooked quinoa
- ¼ cup hummus
- 1 tablespoon lime juice
- ¼ medium avocado, diced
- 3 tablespoons pico de gallo
- 2 tablespoons chopped fresh cilantro

Directions

1. Combine beans and quinoa in a bowl. Stir hummus and lime juice together in a small bowl; thin with water to desired consistency. Drizzle the hummus dressing over the beans and quinoa. Top with avocado, pico de gallo and cilantro.

Prep Time: 10 mins

Total Time: 1 hr 10 mins

Servings: 8

Ingredients

- 1 large head garlic
- ¼ cup extra-virgin olive oil, divided
- ½ cup reduced-fat buttermilk
- 2 ½ teaspoons Dijon mustard
- 1 ½ teaspoons honey
- 1 teaspoon grated lemon zest
- 2 tablespoons lemon juice
- ½ teaspoon onion powder
- ¼ teaspoon salt

Directions

1. Preheat oven to 400°F. Trim and discard top 1/2 inch from garlic head. Place the garlic, cut-side up, on a sheet of foil; drizzle with 1 tablespoon oil. Wrap tightly in the foil; roast until the cloves are completely softened and jammy, about 40

minutes. Let cool for 15 minutes. Squeeze the garlic cloves onto a cutting board; discard garlic skins. Using the flat side of a chef's knife, mash the garlic into a paste.

2. Transfer the garlic paste to a lidded jar or medium bowl. Add buttermilk, mustard, honey, lemon zest, lemon juice, onion powder, salt and the remaining 3 tablespoons oil. Seal the jar and shake, or whisk vigorously in the bowl, until well combined. Shake or whisk before serving.

26. Garlic-Butter Salmon Bites

Prep Time: 15 mins

Total Time: 30 mins

Servings: 4

Ingredients

- 2 tablespoons unsalted butter, melted
- 1 tablespoon lemon juice
- 2 teaspoons grated garlic
- ¼ teaspoon salt
- ¼ teaspoon ground pepper
- 1 pound center-cut salmon fillet, skinned and cut into 1-inch pieces
- Chopped fresh herbs, such as parsley or basil, for garnish

Directions

1. Combine butter, lemon juice, garlic, salt and pepper in a medium bowl. Add salmon pieces and toss to coat well. Let marinate at room temperature for 15 minutes.

2. Preheat broiler to high. Place the salmon pieces on a rimmed baking sheet. Drizzle any remaining marinade from the bowl over the salmon. (If the butter has solidified, microwave for 3 to 5 seconds to warm.) Broil the salmon 4 inches from the heat source until just cooked through, 4 to 5 minutes. Sprinkle with fresh herbs, if desired.

27. Fruit & Yogurt Smoothie

Prep Time: 10 mins

Total Time: 10 mins

Servings: 1

Ingredients

- 3/4 cup nonfat plain yogurt
- 1/2 cup 100% pure fruit juice
- 1 1/2 cups (6 1/2 ounces) frozen fruit, such as blueberries, raspberries, pineapple or peaches

Directions

1. Puree yogurt with juice in a blender until smooth. With the motor running, add fruit through the hole in the lid and continue to puree until smooth.

28. Sheet-Pan Chicken Fajita Bowls

Prep Time: 20 mins

Total Time: 40 mins

Servings: 4

Ingredients

- 2 teaspoons chili powder
- 2 teaspoons ground cumin
- ¾ teaspoon salt, divided
- ½ teaspoon garlic powder
- ½ teaspoon smoked paprika
- ¼ teaspoon ground pepper
- 2 tablespoons olive oil, divided
- 1 ¼ pounds chicken tenders
- 1 medium yellow onion, sliced
- 1 medium red bell pepper, sliced
- 1 medium green bell pepper, sliced
- 4 cups chopped stemmed kale
- 1 (15 ounce) can no-salt-added black beans, rinsed
- ¼ cup low-fat plain Greek yogurt
- 1 tablespoon lime juice
- 2 teaspoons water

Directions

1. Place a large rimmed baking sheet in the oven; preheat to 425 degrees F.

2. Combine chili powder, cumin, 1/2 tsp. salt, garlic powder, paprika, and ground pepper in a large bowl. Transfer 1 tsp. of the spice mixture to a medium bowl and set aside. Whisk 1 Tbsp. oil into the remaining spice mixture in the large bowl. Add chicken, onion, and red and green bell peppers; toss to coat.

3. Remove the pan from the oven; coat with cooking spray. Spread the chicken mixture in an even layer on the pan. Roast for 15 minutes.

4. Meanwhile, combine kale and black beans with the remaining 1/4 tsp. salt and 1 Tbsp. olive oil in a large bowl; toss to coat.

5. Remove the pan from the oven. Stir the chicken and vegetables. Spread kale and beans evenly over the top. Roast until the chicken is cooked through and the vegetables are tender, 5 to 7 minutes more.

6. Meanwhile, add yogurt, lime juice, and water to the reserved spice mixture; stir to combine.

7. Divide the chicken and vegetable mixture among 4
   bowls. Drizzle with the yogurt dressing and serve.

29. Creamy White Chili with Cream Cheese

Prep Time: 10 mins

Total Time: 25 mins

Servings: 6

Ingredients

- 2 (15 ounce) cans no-salt-added great northern beans, rinsed, divided
- 1 tablespoon canola oil
- 1 pound boneless, skinless chicken thighs, trimmed and cut into bite-size pieces
- 1 ½ cups chopped yellow onion (1 medium)
- ¾ cup chopped celery (2 medium stalks)
- 5 cloves garlic, chopped (2 tablespoons)
- 1 teaspoon ground cumin
- ¼ teaspoon salt
- 3 cups unsalted chicken stock
- 1 (4 ounce) can chopped green chiles
- 4 ounces reduced-fat cream cheese
- ½ cup loosely packed fresh cilantro leaves

Directions

1. Mash 1 cup beans in a small bowl with a whisk or potato masher.

2. Heat oil in a large heavy pot over high heat. Add chicken; cook, turning occasionally, until browned, 4 to 5 minutes. Add onion, celery, garlic, cumin and salt. Cook until the onion is translucent and tender, 4 to 5 minutes.

3. Add the remaining whole beans, the mashed beans, stock and chiles. Bring to a boil. Reduce heat to medium and simmer until the chicken is cooked through, about 3 minutes. Remove from heat; stir in cream cheese until melted. Serve topped with cilantro.

30. Slow-Cooker Mediterranean Diet Stew

Prep Time: 15 mins

Total Time: 6 hrs 45 mins

Servings: 6

Ingredients

- 2 (14 ounce) cans no-salt-added fire-roasted diced tomatoes
- 3 cups low-sodium vegetable broth
- 1 cup coarsely chopped onion
- ¾ cup chopped carrot
- 4 cloves garlic, minced
- 1 teaspoon dried oregano
- ¾ teaspoon salt
- ½ teaspoon crushed red pepper
- ¼ teaspoon ground pepper
- 1 (15 ounce) can no-salt-added chickpeas, rinsed, divided
- 1 bunch lacinato kale, stemmed and chopped (about 8 cups)
- 1 tablespoon lemon juice
- 3 tablespoons extra-virgin olive oil

- Fresh basil leaves, torn if large

- 6 lemon wedges

Directions

1. Combine tomatoes, broth, onion, carrot, garlic, oregano, salt, crushed red pepper and pepper in a 4-quart slow cooker. Cover and cook on Low for 6 hours.

2. Measure 1/4 cup of the cooking liquid from the slow cooker into a small bowl. Add 2 tablespoons chickpeas; mash with a fork until smooth.

3. Add the mashed chickpeas, kale, lemon juice and remaining whole chickpeas to the mixture in the slow cooker. Stir to combine. Cover and cook on Low until the kale is tender, about 30 minutes.

4. Ladle the stew evenly into 6 bowls; drizzle with oil. Garnish with basil. Serve with lemon wedges, if desired.